CONTENTS

EMMANUEL LUBANGAKENE

HOW HONEY SAVED MY LIFE

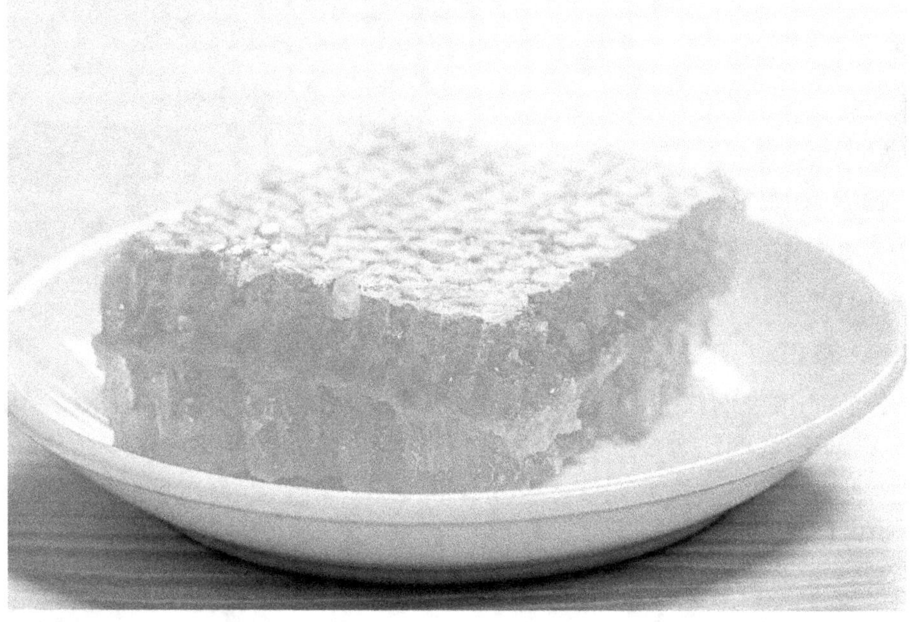

Get to know and Discover the unimaginable Power of honey.

CONTENTS

DISCLAIMER:

The following book, collectively referred to as "ASTHMA THE CURE," is the result of the author's own experience, research, and expression. The purpose of this disclaimer is to outline certain legal and ethical considerations for readers and users of the Book.

1. Accuracy of Information:

While the author has made efforts to ensure the accuracy and reliability of any information presented in the Book, readers are encouraged to verify any factual information independently.

2. Personal Opinions:

Opinions expressed within the Book, whether through characters, narrative, or dialogue, are those of the author and do not necessarily reflect the views of any real individuals, organizations, or entities mentioned.

3. Content Warning:

The Book may contain content that some readers may find offensive, sensitive, or inappropriate. The author acknowledges the diverse sensibilities of readers and advises discretion. Readers are encouraged to assess their comfort level with the content before proceeding.

4. External Links:

Any references or links provided in the Book to external websites, resources, or third-party content are for informational purposes only. The author does not endorse or take responsibility for the accuracy, relevance, or content of external sources.

5. Copyright and Intellectual Property:

The Book is the intellectual property of the author, and all rights are reserved. No part of this Book may be reproduced, distributed, or transmitted in any form or by any means without the prior written permission of the author.

6. Legal:

The author does not take responsibility for Any legal disputes arising from the use or interpretation of the Book.

By accessing, reading, or using the Book, the reader acknowledges and agrees to the terms and conditions outlined in this disclaimer. The author reserves the right to update or modify this disclaimer as necessary.

INTRODUCTION

IT IS OUR REAL LIFE EXPERIENCES AND POSITIVE RESULTS THAT HELP US MAKE BETTER DECISIONS ON OUR HEALTH AND WELLBEING.

Each twist and turn of life's journey reveals vibrant hues that shape the fabric of our existence.

Within this vivid tapestry lies a narrative of personal health struggles, a narrative that traverses the valleys of despair and ascends to the peaks of resilience. At the heart of this transformative odyssey is an unexpected hero –**HONEY**, a golden remedy with unimaginable Power that wove itself into the fabric of my healing journey, coloring every chapter with its sweet and profound influence.

In the following pages, I invite you to embark on a voyage through the labyrinth of my health challenges, a journey illuminated by the golden glow of honey's remarkable and powerful properties.

What began as a quest for relief evolved into a profound exploration of nature's healing wonders, with honey emerging as the ultimate and one of the most powerful natural remedies available to man, offering not just sweetness but a catalyst for transformation.

This is more than a tale of overcoming adversity; it is a testament to the extraordinary power embedded in the simplicity of nature's gifts. Join me as I share the intimate details of my struggles, the pivotal moments of revelation, and the sweet symphony of healing that unfolded when honey became the compass guiding me toward wellness. "Healing Hues" is not just a narrative; it's an exploration of the symbiotic dance between personal challenges and the transformative POWER of a humble jar of honey.

CHAPTER 1: A SWEET SAVIOR

- **Introduction:**

I NEVER KNEW I HAD A GLUTEN PROBLEM, UNTIL I STOPPED EATING HONEY.

The message above is a testimony of the power that honey possesses.
Honey fought for me.
Honey constantly healed me
Honey boosted my immunity and kept it strong

LOOKING BACK,
I NOW SEE THAT IT WAS ONLY IN THE SEASONS WHEN WE DIDN'T HAVE FRESH HONEY COMING IN, THAT I HAD THE MOST ASTHMA ATTACKS.
WHEN I MOVED TO EUROPE AND STOPPED CONSUMING HONEY, GUESS WHAT HAPPENED.

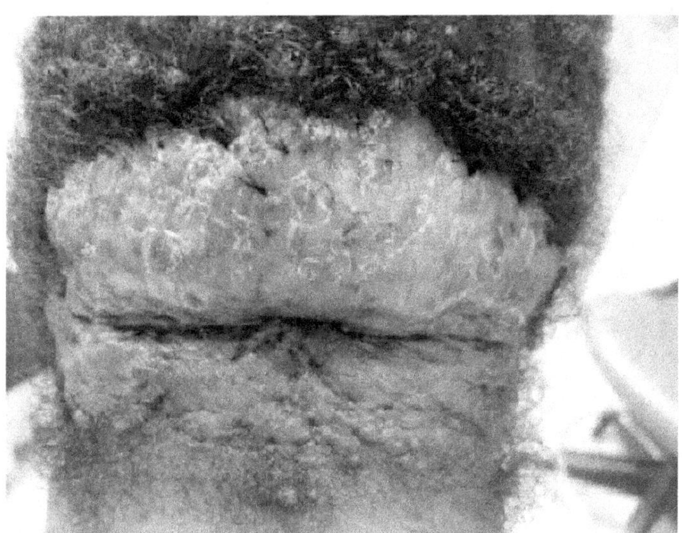

Looking at this image, you will know what I mean by the Power of honey.

My question to you is!

Does that image look pretty?

I guess the answer is no.

If consuming honey regularly prevented that from happening to me, What do you think honey can do for you, In managing your health problems?

- **Turning Point:**

My father was a passionate beekeeper.

He also ran a training center where he held bee classes and trained people how to keep bees. His goals were simple. Passion, teaching people how to make money keeping bees, and lastly, help protect the environment from destruction through keeping bees.

This brief history shows, I grew up always eating fresh Natural pure honey. Even when the honey season would end, we still had a store full of honey to enjoy for the rest of the months, as long as it wasn't all sold out.

I got to know that Honey comes in Different colors, flavors, tastes and after effects.

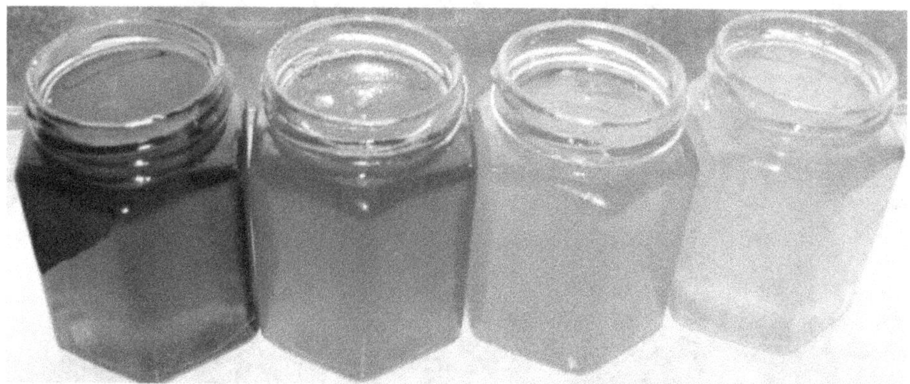

Light white, golden, brown, Dark etc. What determines the color, taste and flavor of honey is the flower from which the nectar is collected by honey bees. Each of these honey varieties has a name(They normally go with the name of the flower from which the honey is from, e.g clover honey, acacia honey etc)..

You would be able to eat as much as you wanted of a certain type during the day, and still be able to have more, while other types were so strong that you only had a few spoonfuls and the body wouldn't take anymore.

I remember a certain type of honey That tasted like milky caramel or Cadbury Eclairs Chocolate. It was so good and flavorful that you just wanted to have more and more of it.

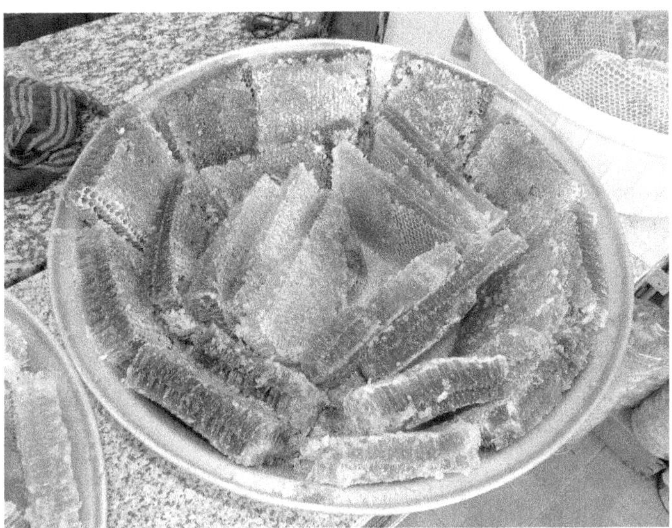

caramel brown sealed comb honey

But it was so strong that the Body couldn't handle much of it. If you were to have a lot of it, you would vomit it out.

Then there was a type that was white, and whenever you would have some, it had a cold sensation in your mouth and just melted away, you could also never have enough of this kind of honey.

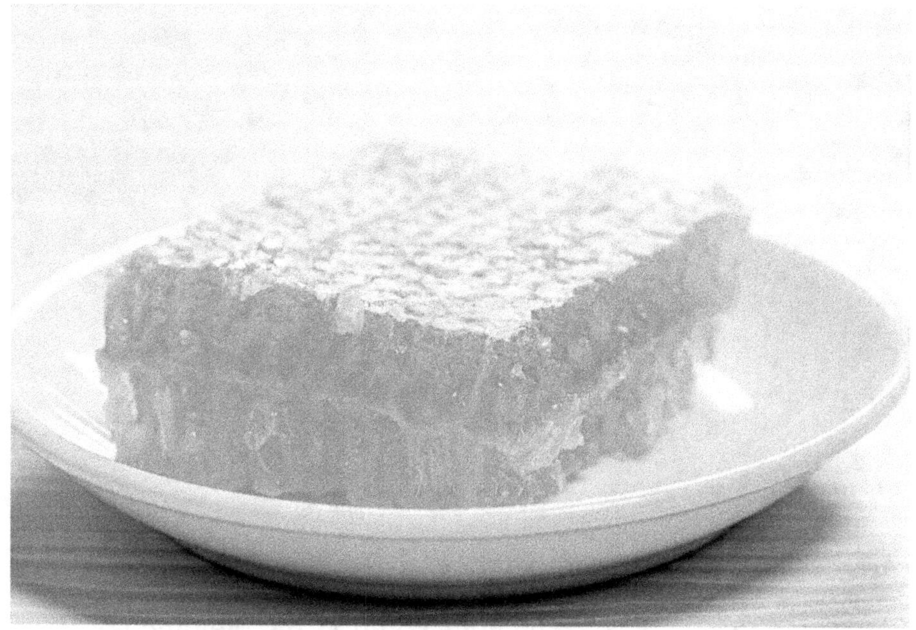

white sealed comb honey comb

This had no after effect so you could eat as much as you wanted without vomiting. I would have many clients coming in only for this Special type. I never had enough of it because it sold out very fast during the honey season.

At a young age, I was diagnosed with asthma. I now see that it was in the months when fresh honey wasn't coming in and I wasn't consuming it regularly, that I had the most asthma attacks. But then the little I was consuming even if not regularly was doing great work in keeping me well even as I was unknowingly consuming what was hurting my body.(gluten).

It was not until I left My Country Uganda in Africa, to live in Europe, and stopped consuming honey that my health condition got really worse.

I was falling sick almost every week.

My Asthma became worse, My eyesight became bad. I would blow my nose till blood came out. My looks became terrible, I got very huge and bad looking pimples on my face that never disappeared. My lips got red, and everyone was worried about me. I didn't know what was going on. I thought it was the change in weather conditions but no. Many pointed to working a lot being the cause of my health problems. They were wrong.

- **The Journey Begins:** My initial experiences with the Healing Power of honey.

I could never imagine that most of my health problems were caused by gluten and Wheat

Honey played a very big role and did a great job in preventing the damage that was being caused by the gluten and wheat I was eating from destroying my health, body and appearance.

Gluten can cause very serious damage and issues to the people whose bodies react to it.

I used to think the term gluten free was a joke, and the people who had problems with gluten pretenders. Little did I know, I had the same problem, and it was the honey I was consuming Daily that was taking all the hits.

Honey is like the greatest Shield against diseases and health conditions.

Amongst the Problems caused by gluten and wheat are:

Acne keloidalis Nuchae

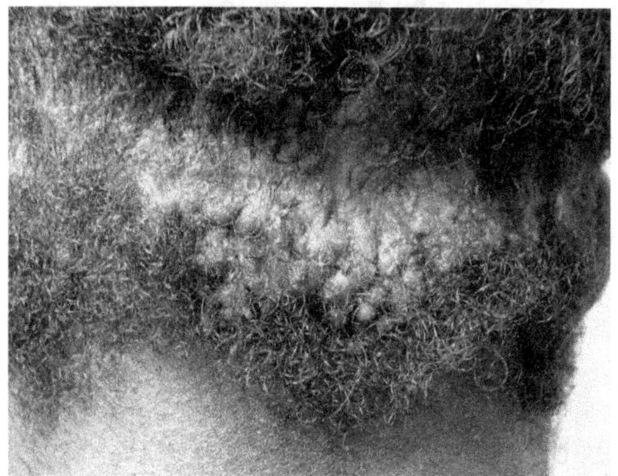

You can see how serious this is. Don't play with gluten. It's not a joking issue.

Asthma

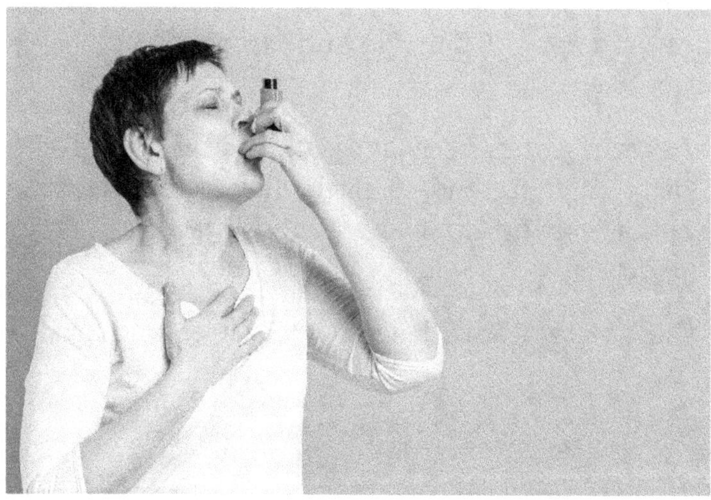

Coeliac disease

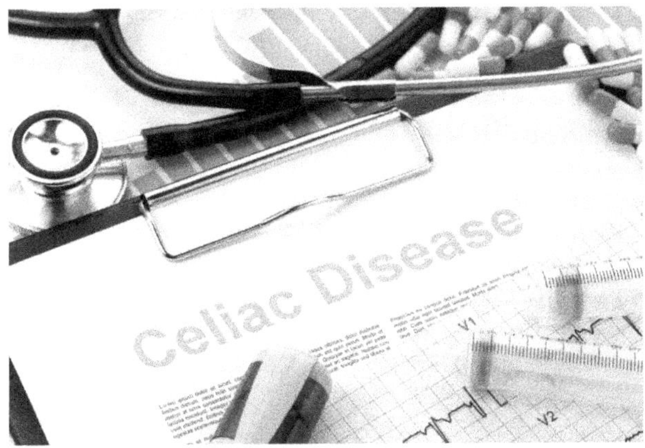

Skin problems and Many others

Not only that, I was falling sick almost every month until I learned that gluten and wheat were the cause of all my health problems.

At the time when I consumed honey, none of the complications I just mentioned appeared nor had much effect on me. I had no other health complications apart from mild asthma attacks that came only at the times when we didn't have honey coming in.

I was also consuming gluten and wheat before I moved to europe. but at the time when honey was regular for me, I never even came close to any symptoms of acne keloidalis nuchae. There was only one time when a small papule appeared on the back of my head but quickly and simply vanished.

Think of all the health problems we have today, and how honey can be used to prevent, heal, preserve and cure.

Sometimes we just can't avoid or prevent ourselves from consuming foods and using products that cause harm and damage to our bodies.

Many times we do it unknowingly. There are so many products and the negative effects of some may appear only after a long time, so we need something in the system that helps fight off that damage. that something is honey.

I used what happened to me as an example of what pure honey can do if you consume it regularly.

CHAPTER 2: THE POWER OF HONEY

- **The Transformative Power:**

Here I delve into the curing Power and specific ways honey boosts immunity and prevents complications, while relating to my experience with Acne keloidalis nuchae, Asthma and other health related problems.

Let's get things Straight. Honey Does Cure. According to my experience, Many Health problems also have a cause(Just like my experience with gluten).

Most causes to our health related issues come from the things we eat, gluten, wheat, sugar, and many dangerous chemicals in products. The list goes on. Many times we consume these products unknowingly.

You can't expect Honey to heal you completely, If the thing causing you health problems is constantly present in your system. All Honey can do with its Powerful properties is to keep The damage at bay. Honey will create a shield and a buffer to prevent more damage, by working around the clock to counteract the damage being caused.

I think the Idea of healing for many is this. I have a gluten problem, and I expect to use Honey's healing Power to make me not have a gluten problem anymore, so that I can continue eating my gluten foods. This doesn't make sense especially when you know that gluten is the one causing you problems.

But they also forget that we as people may have the same blood, but we all have different blood groups. In short, our bodies react differently to different foods and substances. Some people's bodies are more resilient than others.Everyone has a strength of their own. What one person likes, Is not what another desires. It is time we accept reality, that if something is not made for you, it's not. If gluten is not good for you, then don't eat gluten. Honey can help you consume gluten by keeping its effects down, but this only puts more stress on your Body. So why not use it rather to boost your immunity and protect you from other diseases.

This Is exactly what honey was doing for me. I never saw or had any symptoms of acne keloidalis nuchae because I was always consuming Honey. My Asthma was mild because I was consuming Honey. My skin had great healing ability, Because I was Consuming Honey. Gluten and wheat had very little effect on me because I was regularly consuming Honey.

My ratio for consumption of Gluten foods to Honey was 40% Gluten : 60%HONEY respectively. Gluten had no chance . Acne had no chance of developing. TRUST ME, I had a lot of honey that time. We were beekeepers right? Now imagine if I had taken the gluten out, and just had honey and a gluten free diet. this means i would never fall sick ever. my immunity would be so strong, I would be the healthiest man on earth.

My point is that, for honey to manifest its full power and potential in making your health better, first you need honey regularly(but this is not hard to achieve. just replace sugar with honey). Second, you need to understand the cause of your health condition.

AN EXAMPLE IS MY PROBLEM. GLUTEN WAS CAUSING ME THE HEALTH ISSUES. BUT HONEY PREVENTED THE DAMAGE. AFTER TAKING OUT THE GLUTEN, I GET BACK TO HONEY AND MY BODY COMPLETELY HEALS. I AM STRONGER AND HEALTHIER THAN EVER.

Honey's great Healing power works around the clock to

counteract the effects and damage caused to our bodies by products that are not good for our consumption.

Diet and nutrition are very serious issues. We normally don't take them seriously until it's too late.

HONEY'S healing process is a natural one and can only be realized after some time. it took me three years away from consuming honey to realize that it was honey keeping me healthy all along

Such a discovery is not common. But it happened to me, that's why I was able to write this book. I can't say I ate more honey than anyone else on the earth, this I could be wrong, cause there might be someone else somewhere who has a similar privilege of having as much honey as I did.

All I can say is that growing up in a home that sold honey for a living, I sure had a lot of raw natural pure honey around me always. Not only that, I also worked as the man who takes the honey out of the combs and puts it in jars. All day long, I was throwing chunks of comb honey in my mouth and I loved it. I knew exactly what type of honey wouldn't make me vomit, so I would enjoy it all day everyday. I miss those days.

That's why I am on a mission to start the greatest pure natural honey project. Feel free to reach out to me through the links provided at the end of the book If you would like to support me on this journey.

But from experience, I know that If we are to consume as much honey as we do Sugar, the world will be a better place. A great percentage of people would be healthy.

How Honey works within

Honey exhibits strong antioxidant, antimicrobial, anti-inflammatory, antiproliferative, anticancer, and antimetastatic activity..

How do all these properties of honey Cure our diseases?

- **Antioxidant**

A diet high in antioxidants may reduce the risk of many diseases (including heart disease and certain cancers). Antioxidants scavenge free radicals from the body cells and prevent or reduce the damage caused by oxidation. This explains how honey was reducing the risks posed by consuming gluten.

Harnessing Honey's Antioxidant Power

Honey, often praised for its sweet taste and diverse uses, holds a remarkable quality: its potent antioxidant properties. Antioxidants are compounds that counteract oxidative stress in the body, which can lead to cellular damage and contribute to various health issues, including chronic diseases such as cancer and heart disease.

At the heart of honey's antioxidant prowess are its rich array of phytochemicals, including flavonoids, phenolic acids, and enzymes. These bioactive compounds work synergistically to neutralize harmful free radicals, unstable molecules that can wreak havoc on cells by stealing electrons, thereby triggering chain reactions of oxidative damage.

Flavonoids, abundant in honey, are particularly noteworthy for their antioxidant activity. These compounds scavenge free radicals, preventing them from causing cellular harm. Additionally, phenolic acids present in honey play a crucial role in bolstering its antioxidant defense by chelating metal ions, which can catalyze the production of free radicals.

Moreover, the enzymatic activity in honey, notably from glucose oxidase, contributes to its antioxidant potency. Glucose oxidase catalyzes the conversion of glucose to gluconic acid and hydrogen peroxide, the latter of which exhibits antimicrobial and antioxidant properties.

In essence, honey acts as a natural shield against oxidative stress, safeguarding cells and tissues from damage induced by free radicals. By incorporating honey into your diet, you not only savor its delectable sweetness but also fortify your body with a potent arsenal of antioxidants, promoting overall health and well-being.

- **Antimicrobial**

Honey's Antimicrobial Might

Beyond its taste and antioxidant capability, honey stands as a formidable antimicrobial agent, respected for its ability to combat a spectrum of pathogens, including bacteria, fungi, and even certain viruses. This remarkable trait has earned honey a revered status throughout history, as it has been utilized for centuries as a natural remedy for wound healing and infection prevention.

The antimicrobial action of honey is attributed to various factors, chief among them being its low water activity and acidic pH.

Honey's low water content creates an inhospitable environment for microbial growth, effectively dehydrating bacteria and inhibiting their proliferation. Additionally, honey's acidic pH, typically ranging from 3.2 to 4.5, further impedes microbial survival and replication, creating a hostile milieu for pathogens.

Moreover, honey's rich composition of sugars, predominantly glucose and fructose, plays a pivotal role in its antimicrobial efficacy. These sugars exert an osmotic effect, drawing moisture from microbial cells and desiccating them, ultimately leading to their demise. Furthermore, certain types of honey boast unique antimicrobial compounds like methylglyoxal (MGO) and hydrogen peroxide, which amplify their antimicrobial potency.

Furthermore, honey contains an array of bioactive compounds, including hydrogen peroxide, flavonoids, phenolic acids, and bee-derived peptides, all of which contribute to its antimicrobial activity. Hydrogen peroxide, generated enzymatically in honey through the action of glucose oxidase, exhibits broad-spectrum antimicrobial properties, effectively targeting and neutralizing pathogens.

In essence, honey serves as nature's own antimicrobial powerhouse, offering a multifaceted approach to combat microbial threats. Whether applied topically to wounds or consumed internally, honey's antimicrobial prowess serves as a testament to its enduring therapeutic value, providing both ancient wisdom and modern science with a potent ally in the fight against infections.

When it comes to healing, honey plays it part. But remember the part about us consuming things that cause harm to our bodies. As much as you could be using honey to heal, you could at the same time be fighting against HONEY'S ability to heal you fast, by consuming more of the things that damage and weaken your body.

You also need to play a part in understanding what products cause you harm, and avoid them to let Honey work at its maximum potential in Healing you. Also remember, It works best when you consume it regularly. Make Honey your one and only sweetener. And when you grow old, you won't have to deal with health problems that appear over time.

- **Anti-inflammatory**

In addition, honey boasts potent anti-inflammatory properties, making it a cherished ally in the quest for wellness and vitality. Inflammation, a natural response of the immune system to injury or infection, can spiral out of control, leading to chronic diseases such as arthritis, heart disease, and even certain cancers. Honey, with its diverse array of bioactive compounds, emerges as a natural remedy to quell inflammation and promote healing.

Central to honey's anti-inflammatory prowess are its rich content of antioxidants, particularly flavonoids and phenolic acids. These phytochemicals scavenge free radicals and suppress the production of pro-inflammatory cytokines, molecules that orchestrate the inflammatory response. By neutralizing oxidative stress and dampening inflammation, honey helps mitigate tissue damage and promote recovery.

Furthermore, honey's low pH and acidic nature contribute to its anti-inflammatory effect. The acidic environment created by honey inhibits the activity of enzymes involved in the production of inflammatory mediators, thereby attenuating the inflammatory cascade. Additionally, honey's high sugar content exerts an osmotic effect, drawing fluid away from inflamed tissues and reducing swelling.

Moreover, certain types of honey, such as Manuka honey, exhibit enhanced anti-inflammatory properties attributed to unique bioactive compounds like methylglyoxal (MGO) and bee-derived peptides. MGO, in particular, has been shown to inhibit the activity of inflammatory enzymes and modulate immune responses, offering targeted relief from inflammation.

By incorporating honey into your daily regimen, whether as a sweetener in beverages or as a topical application for skin conditions, you harness the power of nature's anti-inflammatory . With its multifaceted approach to inflammation management, honey emerges as a holistic remedy, offering relief and rejuvenation for body and mind.

Just to emphasize on this, regular use of Honey, produces the desired results.
No one has the time to test this out. I have already done the testing, that's why you are reading this book. All you need is to start consuming the right honey, and you will be ok.

- **Antibacterial Wonder:** Explore honey's antibacterial qualities and their impact on health.

Honey's reputation as a potent antibacterial agent is deeply rooted in both ancient tradition and modern scientific inquiry. Across civilizations and centuries, honey has been revered for its ability to combat bacterial infections, offering a natural remedy that stands the test of time. Through a combination of unique properties and bioactive compounds, honey emerges as a formidable force against bacterial pathogens, showcasing its prowess as a true antibacterial wonder.

At the forefront of honey's antibacterial efficacy lies its low moisture content and high sugar concentration. These characteristics create an inhospitable environment for bacterial growth, effectively dehydrating microbes and impeding their ability to thrive. Furthermore, honey's acidic pH, typically ranging from 3.2 to 4.5, creates an additional barrier to bacterial survival, further suppressing their proliferation.

Moreover, honey boasts a rich repertoire of bioactive compounds that contribute to its antibacterial activity. Hydrogen peroxide, generated enzymatically through the action of glucose oxidase, serves as a potent antimicrobial agent, targeting a broad spectrum of bacteria. Additionally, certain types of honey, such as Manuka honey, contain unique antibacterial components like methylglyoxal (MGO) and bee-derived peptides, which augment their antibacterial potency.

Furthermore, honey's multifaceted approach to bacterial inhibition extends beyond direct microbial destruction. Certain bioactive compounds in honey, such as flavonoids and phenolic acids, interfere with bacterial cell signaling pathways and disrupt biofilm formation, rendering bacteria more susceptible to eradication by the immune system or other antimicrobial agents.

By harnessing the antibacterial wonders of honey, whether through topical application to wounds or incorporation into dietary regimens, individuals can tap into nature's own defense mechanism against bacterial infections. With its rich history and proven efficacy, honey stands as a timeless testament to the power of natural remedies in combating bacterial threats and promoting overall health and well-being.

- **Nourishing the Skin:**

Here I Discuss how honey contributes to skin health and how honey worked for me in the prevention of the development of acne Keloidalis nuchae, During the time when I was regularly consuming honey.

It can work for you too in the same way.

In the pursuit of radiant, healthy skin, honey emerges as a

cherished ally, offering a wealth of benefits that extend far beyond its delightful sweetness. From its antibacterial and anti-inflammatory properties to its rich array of antioxidants, honey stands as a versatile remedy for promoting skin health and preventing conditions such as acne keloidalis nuchae.

Acne keloidalis nuchae, characterized by the formation of firm, raised scars or bumps on the back of the neck, often arises from chronic inflammation and follicular irritation. While the exact cause of this condition remains elusive, factors such as shaving, ingrown hairs, and bacterial colonization contribute to its development. Fortunately, honey's multifaceted therapeutic properties offer a holistic approach to managing acne keloidalis nuchae and nurturing skin vitality.

Central to honey's efficacy in skin health is its potent antibacterial action. By inhibiting the growth of pathogenic bacteria such as Staphylococcus aureus, honey helps prevent infections and reduces inflammation, thereby mitigating the risk of exacerbating acne keloidalis nuchae lesions. Moreover, honey's low pH and high sugar content create an unfavorable environment for bacterial growth, further enhancing its antibacterial efficacy.

Furthermore, honey's anti-inflammatory properties play a pivotal role in soothing irritated skin and reducing the redness and swelling associated with acne keloidalis nuchae. By modulating inflammatory responses and scavenging free radicals, honey helps alleviate discomfort and promote healing, fostering a healthier skin environment.

Additionally, honey's antioxidant-rich composition serves as a shield against oxidative stress, a key contributor to skin aging and damage. Flavonoids, phenolic acids, and other bioactive compounds in honey neutralize free radicals and protect skin cells from oxidative damage, helping maintain skin elasticity and vitality.

Moreover, honey's humectant properties attract moisture to the skin, keeping it hydrated and supple. This moisture-retaining effect not only enhances skin softness and elasticity but also facilitates the healing process, promoting the resolution of acne keloidalis nuchae lesions and preventing their recurrence.

By incorporating honey into skincare routines, whether through topical applications or dietary consumption, individuals can harness its myriad benefits for promoting skin health and preventing conditions like acne keloidalis nuchae. With its gentle yet powerful nature, honey serves as a natural elixir for nurturing radiant, resilient skin, restoring confidence and vitality with each application.

The Harmonious Symphony of Honey's Benefits

In the realm of natural remedies, few substances rival the multifaceted marvel that is honey. With its healing touch, immune-boosting prowess, and antioxidant shield, honey orchestrates a symphony of benefits that work in perfect harmony to fortify the body's defenses and preserve overall well-being. Yet, the true power of honey lies not just in its individual attributes, but in the seamless integration of these elements, creating a holistic solution that unfolds its effectiveness over time.

At the heart of honey's potency lies its innate ability to heal and protect. As wounds mend, honey's antimicrobial properties fend off harmful pathogens, while its anti-inflammatory action soothes inflammation and promotes tissue regeneration. This dual action not only accelerates healing but also bolsters the body's natural defenses, enhancing resilience against future threats.

Moreover, honey's immune-boosting properties serve as a stalwart defense against invading pathogens. By stimulating the production of immune cells and modulating immune responses, honey primes the body to fend off infections and maintain health. This proactive approach to immunity not only safeguards against acute illnesses but also confers long-term resilience, preserving vitality and well-being.

Additionally, honey's antioxidant arsenal stands as a guardian against the ravages of oxidative stress. As free radicals are neutralized and cellular damage is mitigated, honey helps preserve cellular integrity and forestall the onset of age-related ailments.

This proactive preservation of health underscores the importance of regular honey consumption, as its cumulative effects gradually unveil their full potential over time.

Indeed, the power of honey is not instantaneous but unfolds gradually, like a blooming flower whose beauty deepens with each passing day. Regular consumption of honey nurtures a reservoir of health and vitality, fortifying the body against the myriad challenges of modern life. As nature's own medicine of wellness, honey serves as a reminder of the profound impact that simple, natural remedies can have on our health and longevity.

Why many don't or can't see the Power of honey

Just because you can't see it working, doesn't mean it's not effective. It's working being invisible shows how powerful honey is, in that it goes in so deep and fast, you can't feel it. The workings of honey are natural. And so is all healing. The effectiveness of honey's healing power is seen after a period of time. If you want to see the effectiveness of honey's power, then you have to regularly use it for a certain period of time, let's say at least three months. Then You will see and know that it's more effective in preventing, Curing and healing compared to medication manufactured in a laboratory.

Why many don't know THE POWER OF HONEY is because the workings are within and happen over time. We can't see ourselves growing but we know we are.

Today people just want a fast solution to everything.

Quick relief medication has sold us all into thinking that only medication manufactured in the laboratory is effective.

This is why some people don't even think about Honey as a solution to health problems.

But what they don't want to comprehend is that Quick relief medication manufactured, can also have serious consequences to our health over time. Some may even lead to more serious health problems.

Note: The effectiveness of honey also depends on the type of honey you consume, how much and how regularly you consume it. Remember what I wrote about ratio?, On how much honey you consume to how much of the substances that affect your body you are also consuming.

Just taking a spoon a day, three days a week might have little to do to counteract the two loaves of bread and 20 spoons of sugar you have on a daily basis.

This kind of imbalance makes the power of honey not so effective.

What many expect is to buy a jar today, take a few Spoons and all diseases will disappear. That's not how honey works. It could though if you knew what caused your immunity to be weak. Then take it out and let honey do its job. Even doctors often advise on a certain type of food after prescription of drugs.

We have all been sold into having this mindset that everything needs scientific medication or drugs produced in a laboratory, hospitals and doctors etc. our minds have gone so far that we bypass some simple solutions that actually work.
This kind of mindset has driven us away from the simplicity of things and natural ways that actually cure and heal real diseases, at little or no cost.

I am sick today, I want to get better today, forgetting that the sickness might have also not come right away. it might have been in your system for sometime working its way up .
This kind of I want it now mind has also pushed us away from natural methods that truly heal but need time, to drugs that give quick relief but don't cure.
It means we can keep having the problem, but cover them up with quick relief drugs, which in return can be very dangerous especially for conditions like asthma and others.

I don't blame anyone. I was there too.

Such a discovery like I did needs time to realize. It's only after some time of regularly consuming honey, that you will realize its power.

When we understand how things work, then we can plan our healing way before we even get sick. which means we will never get sick. if we consume honey regularly just as we do with sugar, and take out all the bad foods and substances that cause us health issues, don't you think we will always be healthy?

Mind set **(Not everyone should know.)**

If everyone knew the power of Honey, how it works and how we can all apply it in our daily lives, Then sickness would be very little amongst mankind.

I dont think it's in the interests of the big medication producing companies to tell everyone that just eating honey daily can cure you.

TRUST ME. If they wanted everyone to know that honey has power, posters would be up everywhere. The doctors first question would be, do you take honey, if yes , how much of it.

Letting people know of a permanent or enduring solution and cure for disease would be bad for business.
the truth is that there are conditions that don't have a cure yet, but there are those with known cures, yet the information is not available to the public

Just like asthma. If everyone got cured today, the inhaler factory would suffer loss. it's the fact.

Another problem is we the people ourselves, don't take warnings to health seriously until it's too late

UNTIL THAT ACNE FORMS IN THE BACK OF YOUR HEAD, YOU WONT STOP MUNCHING DOWN ALL THE FAST FOOD FILLED WITH 90% WHEAT AND GLUTEN.

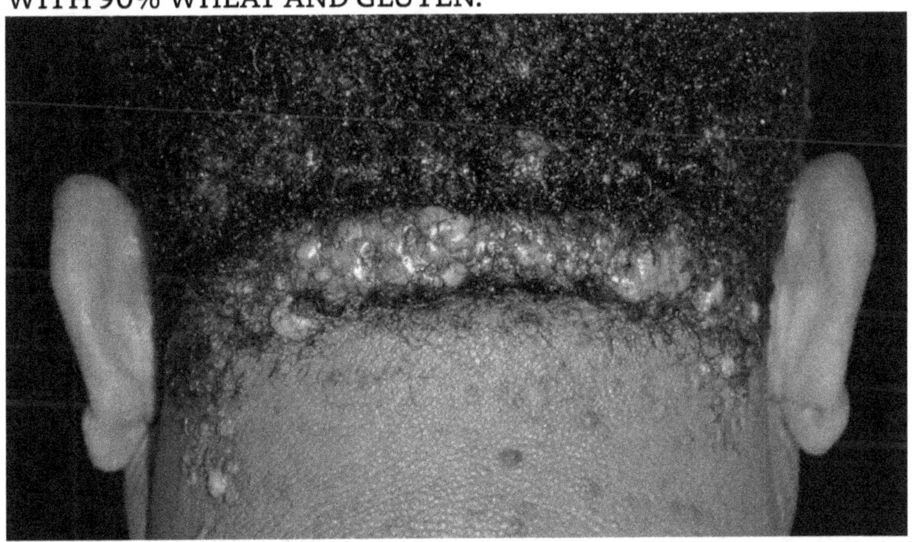

It's only when you see that thing on your head that you start to worry and start taking care. but then if you wait until the damage appears on your head, think about this, how much damage will it have caused already on the inside.

Would it not be cheaper stopping the sugar, reducing the bread and having ¼ a jar of honey a day. rather than wait till its bad then head out for expensive surgery and who knows what the outcome will be.

CHAPTER 3: NOT ALL HONEY POSSESS POWER(THE DARK SIDE OF HONEY)

I mentioned in the beginning about the Power that Honey has.

I would Like to clearly state that not all honey you see, Possesses Power., and not every honey you see is honey

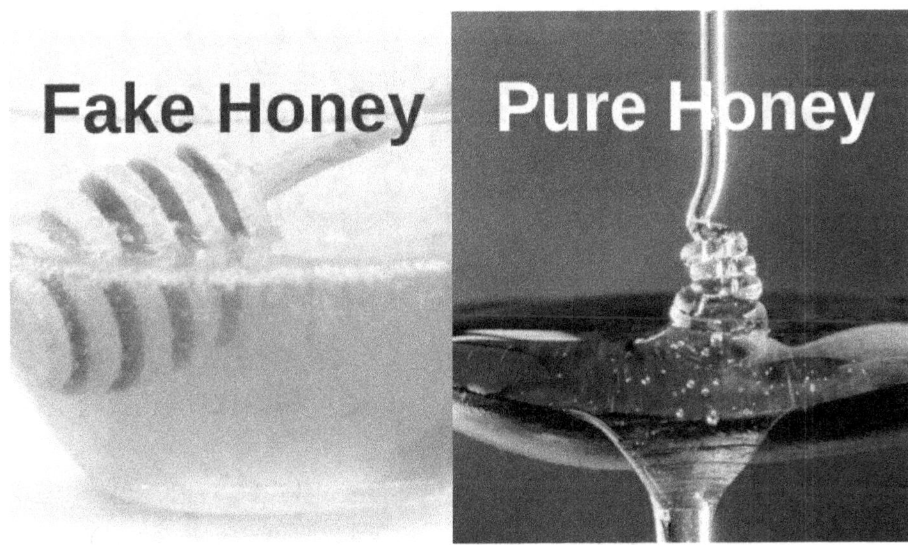

Understanding what real honey is, will both save your money so you don't waste it on a useless product, and also save your health, cause when you buy something sold as honey but it's not, it can

definitely have negative effects on your health.

All fake honey is fake, and not all real honey is real.

The demand for honey is so high,, not only has pure honey been adulterated, it has also led to the manufacture of artificial honey. There are so many circulating videos on life where producers and manufactures are caught red handed packaging false honey.

Leaving the illegals aside, There are those that claim they can manufacture honey. The sad thing is that even artificial honey is sold as Honey.

Fake Honey

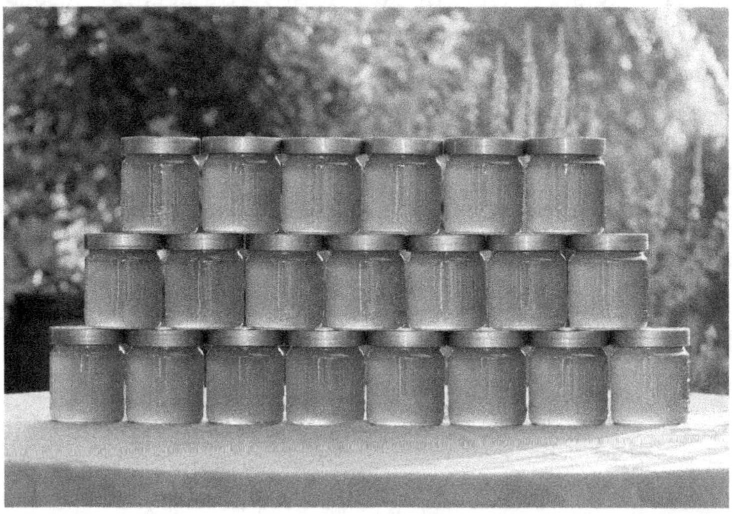

It might look like honey, smell like honey, taste like honey, but it isn't honey. It's poison.

It's sad to say that a huge percentage of honey sold on the market is fake. You might be buying fake honey, and that's why you can't see HONEY'S POWER.

If they wrote, FAKE HONEY clearly on the jar, I don't think real honey buyers would buy it. Fake honey shouldn't even have the name honey on it. Because it's not honey, and doesn't have anything to do with honey. I think the name of honey produced by honey bees needs to changed, because the word Honey can be used for anything these days. Even for sugar.

In the midst of honey's golden allure lies a shadowy impostor lurking in the wings: fake honey. Crafted through deceit and adulteration, fake honey poses a threat to both consumer health and the integrity of the honey industry. This insidious counterfeit undermines the purity and potency of genuine honey, tarnishing its reputation and eroding consumer trust.

Fake honey, often concocted from sugar syrups or diluted with water, lacks the rich array of nutrients and bioactive compounds found in authentic honey. Devoid of the healing touch and immune-boosting prowess of genuine honey, these counterfeit products offer little more than empty calories and false promises.

Moreover, fake honey may harbor harmful contaminants and additives, ranging from antibiotics and heavy metals to artificial flavorings and preservatives. Consuming such adulterated honey not only deprives the body of genuine health benefits but also exposes it to potential risks and adverse effects.

The proliferation of fake honey not only undermines consumer health but also jeopardizes the livelihoods of honest beekeepers and producers. By flooding the market with cheap imitations, counterfeiters undercut the value of genuine honey, driving down prices and eroding profits for those who uphold the highest standards of quality and integrity.

To combat the scourge of fake honey, vigilance and discernment are paramount. Consumers must educate themselves on the telltale signs of counterfeit honey, from unusual clarity and overly sweet taste to suspiciously low prices and dubious origins. By supporting reputable producers and demanding transparency in labeling and sourcing, consumers can safeguard their health and integrity against the menace of fake honey.

Producers of fake honey are everywhere. The demand for honey is very high and supply is very low.

Not all real honey is real

How can real Honey not be real?

- **Adulteration Explained:** Adulteration and the dangers of adulteration in the honey industry.

Beekeeping for honey production is serious business.

The demand for honey Is so high, but the supply is very low, because it takes a lot of work, planning ,investing and many times dealing with losses, for the beekeeper to produce pure natural Honey.

Today's massive Industrial era has also led to the destruction of Nature, which has led to a great decline in the production of natural pure honey. Land with natural vegetation being cleared up to make way for huge monoculture farms reduces the beekeepers potential to produce much honey. Honey bees make honey from nectar that comes from flowers. The less nectar there is, the less honey you will get.

But the demand has just continued to rise because of more and more people getting aware of the benefits of honey . So what are the beekeepers and Honey Suppliers to do?
The honest and passionate ones have continued to persevere,

But many have turned to greed. It is not about health anymore. It is all about meeting the high demand on the market and making profits. Millions of people unknowingly consume what is sold to them as honey in the name of health.

In the world of honey, where golden hues and sweet promises abound, there exists a sinister practice that threatens to taint the purity and integrity of this beloved natural medicine: adulteration. Adulteration of honey involves the addition of cheap fillers, such as sugar syrups or other sweeteners, to deceive consumers and boost profits. While this clandestine practice may seem harmless on the surface, the dangers it poses to both consumer health and the honey industry are profound and far-reaching.

Adulterated honey undermines the very essence of this precious nectar, diluting its nutritional value and therapeutic properties. By substituting high-quality honey with inferior ingredients, adulterators compromise the integrity of the product, robbing consumers of the genuine health benefits and sensory delights that authentic honey offers.

Moreover, the adulteration of honey presents a myriad of health risks and safety concerns. Fake honey may contain harmful contaminants, such as antibiotics, pesticides, and heavy metals, which pose serious threats to consumer health. Additionally, the presence of undisclosed allergens or additives in adulterated honey can trigger adverse reactions and allergic responses in susceptible individuals, further compounding the risks.

Beyond the realm of consumer health, adulteration undermines the sustainability and viability of the honey industry as a whole. By flooding the market with counterfeit products, adulterators drive down prices and undercut honest beekeepers and producers who adhere to stringent quality standards. This not only erodes consumer trust but also jeopardizes the livelihoods of those who depend on the honey industry for their sustenance and livelihood.

To combat the dangers of adulteration in the honey industry, stringent regulations, robust testing protocols, and increased transparency are essential. By holding adulterators accountable for their deceptive practices and enforcing strict penalties for violations, authorities can deter illicit activities and safeguard the integrity of the honey supply chain.

As consumers, it is our responsibility to remain vigilant and discerning in our choices, seeking out reputable producers and authentic honey sources that prioritize quality and transparency. By supporting ethical practices and demanding honesty and integrity in the honey industry, we can protect our health, preserve the purity of honey, and uphold the values of truth and authenticity.

Adulteration is not done by greedy producers alone, but some sneaky beekeepers are in on it too.

The Bitter Truth: Beekeepers and the Deceptive Practice of Self-Adulteration

Amidst the idyllic landscapes where bees labor tirelessly to create nature's golden elixir, a troubling trend has emerged within the ranks of beekeepers: self-adulteration of honey. Faced with environmental degradation and dwindling floral resources, some beekeepers have resorted to artificial means to boost honey production, tarnishing the purity and integrity of this revered natural treasure.

In their quest for higher yields, certain beekeepers have turned to providing bees with sugar syrups and artificial sweeteners, effectively tricking them into producing more honey than they naturally would. This practice, known as self-adulteration, not only compromises the authenticity of the honey but also raises serious ethical and ecological concerns.

By supplementing bee diets with sugar-based solutions, beekeepers disrupt the delicate balance of nature's symbiotic relationship between bees and flowers. Instead of foraging for nectar from a diverse array of floral sources, bees become dependent on artificial substitutes, leading to a loss of biodiversity and genetic diversity within bee populations.

Moreover, self-adulteration perpetuates a vicious cycle of environmental degradation, as the depletion of natural habitats and floral resources continues unabated. Without sufficient floral diversity to sustain bee populations, ecosystems suffer, and the delicate dance of pollination falters, jeopardizing the future of countless plant species and the biodiversity of our planet.

Furthermore, the practice of self-adulteration undermines consumer trust and confidence in the honey industry, as unsuspecting consumers may unknowingly purchase honey that has been artificially manipulated. This deception not only deprives consumers of the genuine health benefits and sensory delights of authentic honey but also erodes the reputation of honest beekeepers who adhere to ethical and sustainable practices.

To address the issue of self-adulteration in the honey industry, greater transparency, accountability, and regulation are urgently needed. By promoting sustainable beekeeping practices, protecting natural habitats, and fostering a culture of integrity and honesty within the industry, we can preserve the purity of honey and safeguard the vital role that bees play in maintaining the health and balance of our planet.

- **Consequences**: potential health consequences of consuming adulterated honey.

Every one that buys honey, pays whatever amount asked for a reason..

The main reasons being Health related. Otherwise, they would just buy Sugar instead, and sweetener was all they needed. After all Sugar is sweet, abundant, and probably cheaper than Honey.

Therefore, whatever you are paying for should be the real deal. But its not.

So as this person(you and me) unknowingly continues consuming this Product that contains Chemicals, Not knowing the they just Might be the same chemicals He/she is running from.

Because They Think it's good for them, and because it's sold in the name of honey yet it's not, They take way too Much of it which in return worsens their health conditions. And because they are convinced that Honey will make them well, They even buy more of it, till they get hospitalized.

This is why we all need to take the things we consume seriously. But then we end up paying the price because of some greedy fellows who only care about profiting.

This kind of activity Is hard to manage, and can only be controlled by the consumers. The power that most consumers lack is knowledge. By knowledge, you make the right decisions, Knowledge gives us the power to know what we want and choose exactly what we need. How, when and where to get it. With the right information, you will understand the right honey to buy, and where to buy it, So that you can enjoy its full benefits in your life.

CHAPTER 4: THE REAL HONEY YOU NEED THAT HAS POWER

To me, real honey that possesses power is honey produced by bees in a natural environment, and the bee keeper or producer has not done anything to manipulate its production.

It doesn't matter what type it is, or from which plant nectar it comes from, All that matters is, it has to be raw, natural and pure. Yes there are some plant nectars that produce honey with stronger flavor than others, but most of the talk about one type of honey being better than another, may have some marketing to do with it. All the honey consumer needs to worry about is if the honey they are buying and consuming is Natural and pure. You may prefer one type over another because of taste and flavor, but any pure natural Honey works just fine. You have seen my story, I know some of the trees from which my honey came. It didn't matter, they all worked for me. There is a lot of buzz going on about manuka honey, but until you taste it as I did and compare it with other honeys it will always just be buzz with a little marketing language in it. I do not know if we have manuka in Africa. It might exist. But it wasn't part of the type of honey I was eating. Yet what I was consuming did an extraordinary job, in keeping that acne away. So to me What matters Is the purity of honey left in its natural form being tampered with.

Real honey that has power, doesn't matter what type of honey it is, or what type of nectar it's from. What matters, and makes it have

POWER is that It's natural raw and pure honey.

A beekeeper's job is basically to manage his/her bee colonies to produce natural honey.

In other words, bring the honey bees closer and help them work in a way that guarantees a honey reward every year. bees are already doing their thing. but if you want to be sure of some honey every honey season, then you have to manage them. That's what bee keeping is. As long as beekeepers don't tamper with the way the bees are making the honey, then you can be sure that it's pure honey you will be getting.

REAL HONEY CRYSTALLIZES

I couldn't help but talk about crystallization

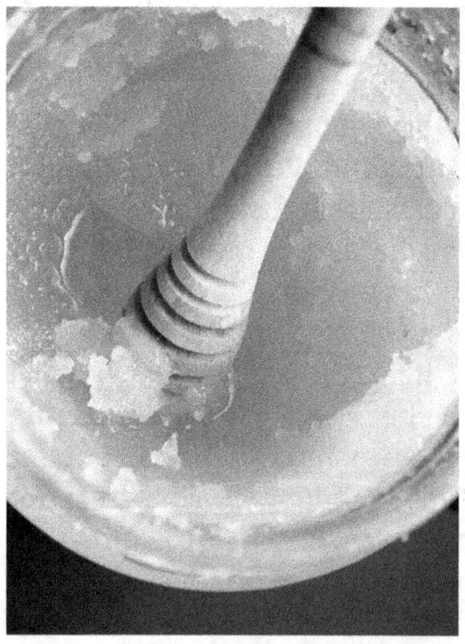

Many people get worried when they wake up and find that their honey has crystallized. Crystallization also drives down sales because many honey buyers are worried thinking there could be sugar added, but it's not. Thankfully, today this book is here to clear up the air.

Understanding Honey Crystallization

In the journey from hive to table, honey may undergo a fascinating transformation known as crystallization. This natural phenomenon occurs when glucose molecules in honey form solid crystals, giving the liquid honey a granulated or "crystallized" texture. While some consumers may find this change concerning, the truth is that honey crystallization is a perfectly natural and reversible process, reflecting the purity and authenticity of the honey.

Crystallization is a hallmark of high-quality honey and is actually a sign of its purity and unadulterated nature. Genuine honey, rich in natural sugars and trace minerals, is more prone to crystallization compared to processed or adulterated honey. The speed and degree of crystallization depend on various factors, including the floral source, temperature, and moisture content of the honey.

Contrary to popular misconceptions, crystallized honey is not spoiled or unsafe to consume. In fact, crystallization preserves the freshness and flavor of honey, locking in its unique aroma and taste. Additionally, crystallized honey tends to have a thicker, spreadable consistency, making it ideal for use as a topping or ingredient in cooking and baking.

Moreover, the crystallization of honey is reversible and can be easily remedied with gentle heating. By placing the container of crystallized honey in a bowl of warm water, the crystals will dissolve, restoring the honey to its liquid state without compromising its quality or nutritional value.

In essence, honey crystallization is a natural and benign process that underscores the authenticity and purity of the honey. Rather than being a cause for concern, consumers can embrace crystallized honey as a testament to its natural origins and enjoy its unique texture and flavor with confidence, knowing that they are savoring a genuine and wholesome product straight from the hive.

CHAPTER 5: HOW TO GET REAL HONEY THAT HAS POWER

GO LOCAL.

Supporting Local Beekeepers

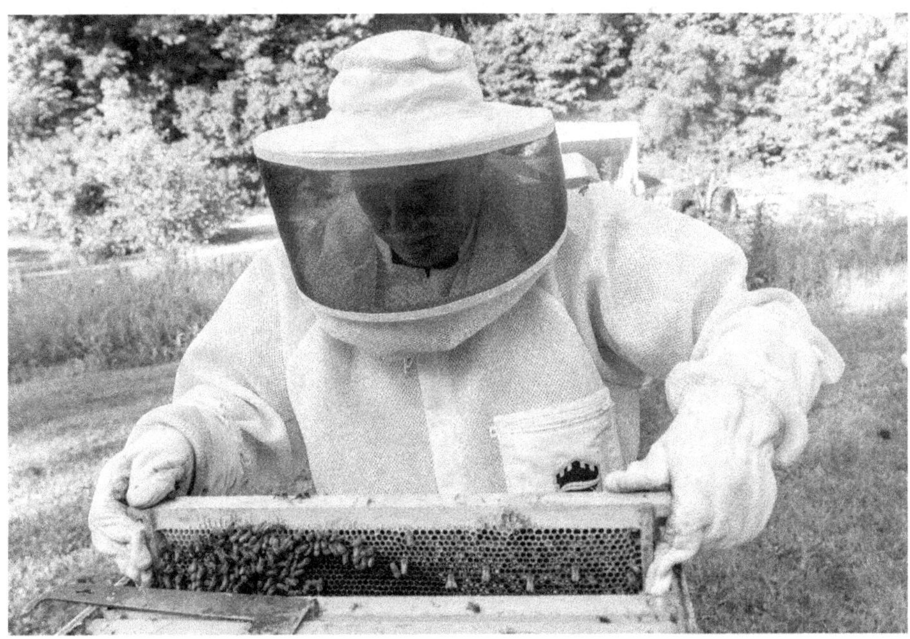

There is always a high chance that the beekeeper next door has the real deal. you will be surprised how many local beekeepers you have around. Going local does not only give you a high chance of getting real honey, but it also helps support the local beekeepers around, which brings them much joy and boosts them to do an even better job in providing pure natural quality honey. knowing that the people around recognise them, makes them also accountable and gets them to do things better for their reputation.

So how do you find the beekeeper next door? You can simply search online for beekeepers associations in your area or close to your area, these always keep track and have information about the beekeepers next door. Which one would you trust? honey imported from a far country or the one hand packed from the beekeeper next door.

Local beekeepers normally also run small honey shops around town, where they sell their own honey, other local beekeepers honey, and many other products that come from honey bees. They normally have fixed locations which means you can create a personal relationship with them to ensure they serve you the real deal. The fixed location means they take their reputation seriously.

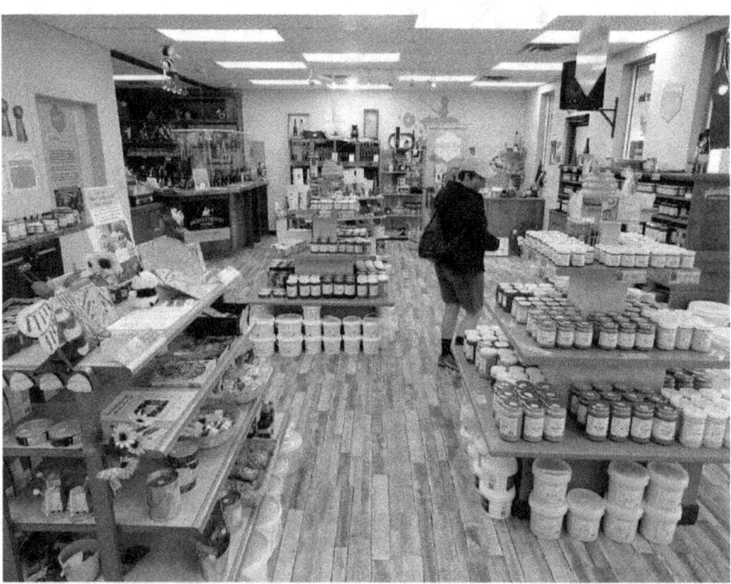

Local bee store

Depending on where you live, not every local beekeeper owns a shop. But they do own bee yards. Most are more than happy to receive visitors to their bee yards and operation, because it can also be an extra source of income. Bee tourism is great for the beekeeper, because people pay for both the visit and their time to show them around and give exciting lectures. Beekeepers love to teach and talk about bees. Most of the time, visitors will leave pure honey in their hands.

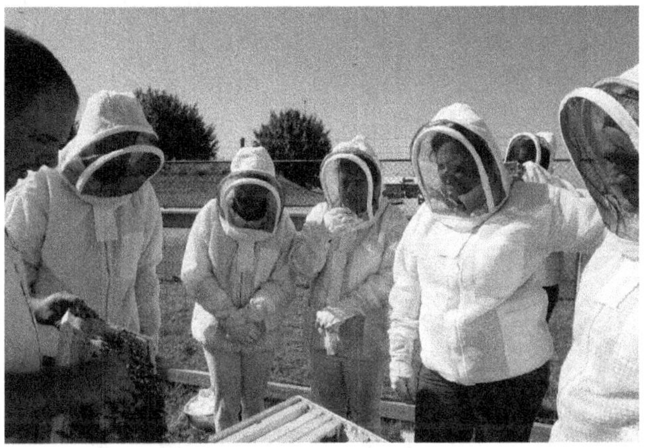

Visiting a bee yard is a great way to learn about honey. You can use this opportunity to create a relationship, get contacts and get supplied with pre natural honey straight off the bee yard.

- **The Ethical Choice:**

Embracing the Buzz: The Ethical and Health Benefits of Local Honey

In a world increasingly defined by mass production and global supply chains, there's something profoundly enriching about connecting with the source of our sustenance on a local level. When it comes to honey, this connection takes on a special significance, offering not just a sweet treat, but a gateway to ethical and healthful living.

Obtaining honey from local beekeepers is a testament to our commitment to ethical consumption and sustainable practices. By supporting local apiarists, we directly contribute to the preservation of bee populations and the health of our ecosystems. Local beekeepers prioritize the well-being of their colonies, employing ethical beekeeping practices that prioritize the health and vitality of their bees and the surrounding environment. This stewardship ensures that the honey we enjoy is not only delicious but also ethically sourced and environmentally responsible.

Beyond its ethical implications, honey from local beekeepers offers a wealth of health benefits that extend far beyond its delectable taste. Local honey is often raw and unprocessed, retaining its natural enzymes, antioxidants, and pollen content. Consuming local honey can help alleviate seasonal allergies by exposing the body to small amounts of local pollen, thereby building immunity and reducing allergy symptoms. Moreover, raw honey contains beneficial enzymes and antioxidants that support immune function, promote digestive health, and contribute to overall well-being.

In essence, obtaining honey from local beekeepers is not just about satisfying our sweet tooth—it's a holistic embrace of ethical consumption and mindful living. By choosing local honey, we nourish our bodies with pure, healthful goodness while supporting the hardworking beekeepers who nurture and protect our precious pollinators. So let's savor the sweetness of local honey and celebrate the ethical and healthful journey it represents.

- **Investing in Health:**

The Sweet Investment: Why Genuine, Local Honey Is Worth Every Penny

In a marketplace flooded with mass-produced alternatives, genuine, local honey stands as a shining beacon of quality, integrity, and unparalleled flavor. While it may come with a slightly higher price tag compared to its store-bought counterparts, the investment in genuine, local honey is one that pays dividends in both taste and value.

First and foremost, genuine, local honey offers a purity and authenticity that cannot be replicated by mass-produced alternatives. Sourced directly from local beekeepers who prioritize ethical and sustainable practices, local honey is a true reflection of its natural origins. Unlike store-bought honey, which may be processed, adulterated, or sourced from unknown origins, local honey is raw and unfiltered, retaining its full complement of nutrients, enzymes, and antioxidants. This purity not only enhances the flavor and richness of the honey but also ensures that we are nourishing our bodies with the highest quality ingredients.

Moreover, the higher cost of genuine, local honey is a reflection of the care, craftsmanship, and dedication that goes into its production. Local beekeepers invest significant time, resources, and expertise in nurturing their bee colonies, harvesting honey, and bringing their products to market. By supporting local beekeepers, we not only contribute to the preservation of bee populations and the health of our ecosystems but also sustain the livelihoods of those who work tirelessly to bring us this golden elixir of nature.

Furthermore, genuine, local honey offers a unique sensory

experience that transcends the ordinary. From its distinct floral notes to its velvety texture and complex flavor profile, local honey captivates the palate and delights the senses in ways that store-bought alternatives simply cannot match. This sensory journey is a testament to the richness and diversity of our natural world, inviting us to savor each spoonful and appreciate the beauty of the bees' labor.

In essence, the higher cost of genuine, local honey is not just a reflection of its superior quality—it's an investment in our health, our communities, and our connection to the natural world. So let's savor the sweetness of local honey and celebrate the abundance of goodness that it brings into our lives.

Buy from backyard beekeeper

A backyard beekeeper is an individual who keeps and manages a small number of honeybee colonies on their residential property, typically in a suburban or rural setting. Unlike commercial beekeepers who operate large-scale apiaries for commercial purposes, backyard beekeepers often maintain bee colonies as a hobby or for personal use, such as pollination of home gardens and production of small quantities of honey for personal consumption or local sale. Backyard beekeepers may manage anywhere from one to a few dozen hives, depending on the size of their property and their level of experience and expertise in beekeeping practices.

You can find Backyard beekeepers with stalls at small local markets or beekeeping conventions that only happen a few times a month or year.

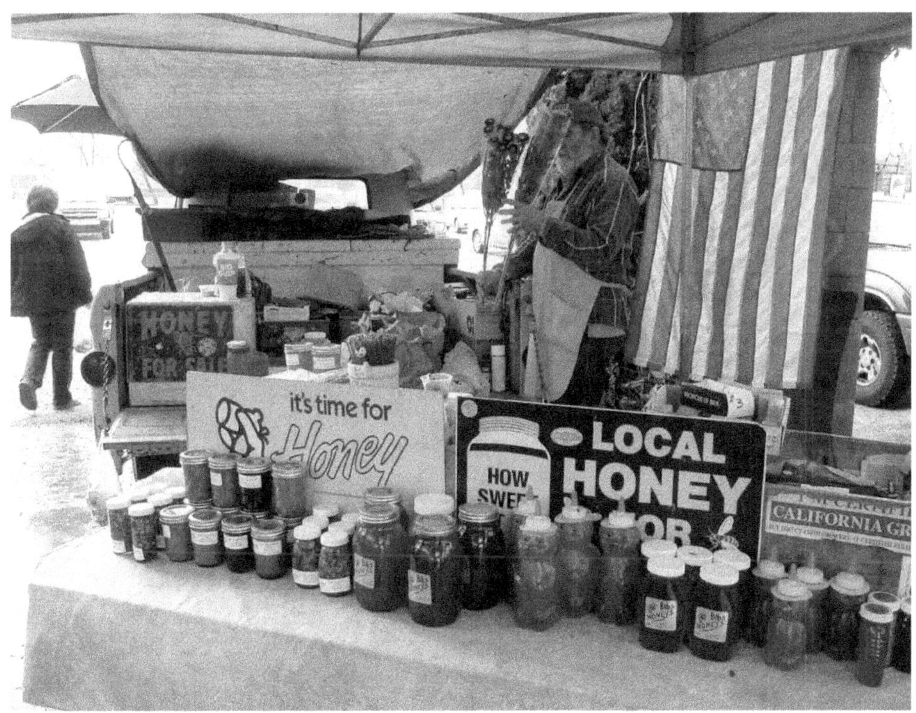

Try beekeeping your self.

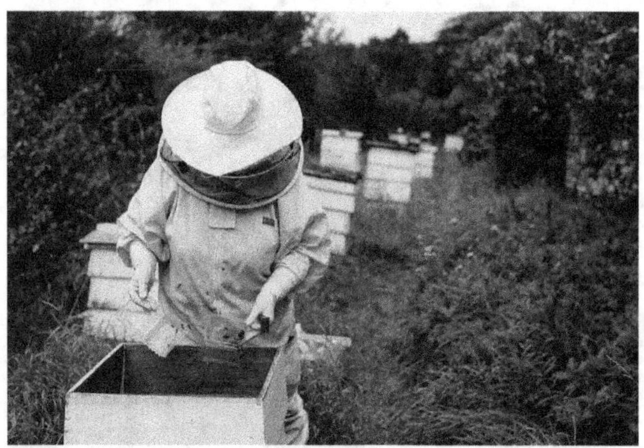

This is not for everyone, but it can be one way, you guarantee you are getting the real thing. Take a bee class, watch bee lecture videos, read some books(There are lots of books, just contact me for links), and learn from the beekeeper next door.

All beginnings are challenging, but once you get the hang of it, you might actually get to love it. It's neither hard nor complicated. If you have got a piece of land in the country somewhere, have a little time and can get over the fear of bees, then you can give beekeeping a try. Doing it just to produce enough honey for yourself to run you through the year is not something difficult.

Lastly, contact local beekeepers in your area and find out if their honey is available on the shelves of your nearest convenience stores. Some local producers of pure honey produce enough honey that they are even able to supply some store chains in your area.

Also make it a point to read what's written on every jar you buy from a store, to make sure you are not being cheated out of your money and health.

CHAPTER 6: SEASONS OF GOLD

- **Understanding Seasons:**

Nature's Sweet Symphony: Understanding the Seasonal Dance of Honey Production

Honey production is a delicate ballet choreographed by the rhythms of nature's seasons, where each stage unfolds with its own unique beauty and significance. Throughout the year, bees diligently gather nectar from blooming flowers, transforming it into the liquid gold we know as honey. Yet, this process is far from constant, as it ebbs and flows in harmony with the changing seasons.

In spring, as the world awakens from its winter slumber, bees emerge from their hives in search of the first blossoms of the season. With an insatiable appetite for nectar, they embark on a frenzied foraging spree, collecting copious amounts of nectar to fuel their growing colonies. Spring is a time of abundance and vitality, as bees work tirelessly to build up their honey stores in preparation for the leaner months ahead.

As summer unfolds, the landscape explodes with color and fragrance, providing a rich tapestry of floral diversity for bees to explore. During this bountiful season, honey production reaches its peak, as bees feast on a profusion of nectar-rich flowers. It is a time of frenetic activity and industriousness, as bees labor tirelessly to fill their honeycombs to capacity, storing away the surplus nectar for the coming winter months.

However, as summer gives way to autumn and the days grow shorter and cooler, the pace of honey production begins to slow. With fewer flowers in bloom and cooler temperatures inhibiting foraging activity, bees focus their efforts on consolidating their resources and preparing their hives for the onset of winter. As the last of the season's blooms fade away, bees retreat into their hives, where they will hunker down and wait out the cold months ahead.

In this seasonal dance of honey production, each stage plays a vital role in the lifecycle of the hive, shaping the quantity and quality of the honey that is ultimately harvested. By understanding and appreciating the seasonal rhythms of honey production, we gain a deeper appreciation for the intricate interplay between bees, flowers, and the natural world around us.

- **Making Pre-Orders:**

Connecting with Local Beekeepers: A Guide to Making Pre-Orders

Making pre-orders from local beekeepers is a wonderful way to support ethical beekeeping practices, enjoy the freshest honey, and forge connections within your community. Here's a step-by-step guide to help you navigate the process and make the most of your local honey experience:

Research Local Beekeepers: Start by researching beekeepers in your area. You can use online directories, social media platforms, or community forums to find beekeepers who sell honey locally.

Reach Out to Beekeepers: Once you've identified potential beekeepers, reach out to them to inquire about their honey availability and pre-order process. Many beekeepers will have contact information listed on their website or social media profiles, or you can reach out through email or phone.

Ask About Pre-Order Options: Inquire about pre-order options and deadlines for placing orders. Some beekeepers may offer pre-ordering for specific honey harvests or seasonal varieties, while others may have ongoing availability.

Place Your Order: Once you've gathered all the necessary information, place your pre-order with the beekeeper. Be sure to specify the quantity and type of honey you'd like, as well as any special instructions or preferences you may have.

Arrange Pickup or Delivery: Coordinate with the beekeeper to arrange pickup or delivery of your honey order. Depending on the beekeeper's preferences and availability, you may be able to pick up your order directly from their apiary or arrange for delivery to your home or a designated pickup location.

Enjoy Your Local Honey: Once you've received your honey order, take the time to savor its unique flavors and aromas. Local honey offers a taste of your region's biodiversity and a connection to the natural world around you. Use it in your favorite recipes, drizzle it over yogurt or toast, or simply enjoy it by the spoonful.

By making pre-orders from local beekeepers, you not only support sustainable beekeeping practices and local economies but also gain access to the freshest, most flavorful honey your region has to offer. So go ahead, reach out to your local beekeepers, and embark on a sweet journey of connection and community through the golden goodness of local honey.

The safest honey you can buy is comb honey(This is only if you don't trust the beekeeper, and have a little time to take the honey out of the combs yourself. Trust me, it is neither hard nor complicated) in . Most of the time comb honey can only be obtained directly from the beekeeper. Sometimes you can buy your honey while still in combs and pay the beekeeper extra to extract it as you watch. This works if you are buying in bulk to have enough honey for the rest of the year.

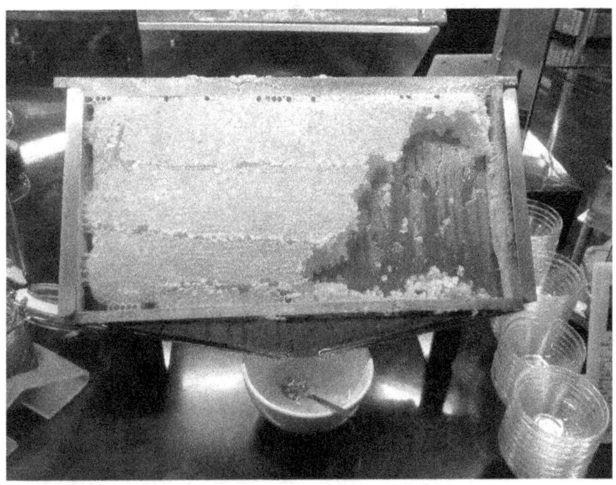

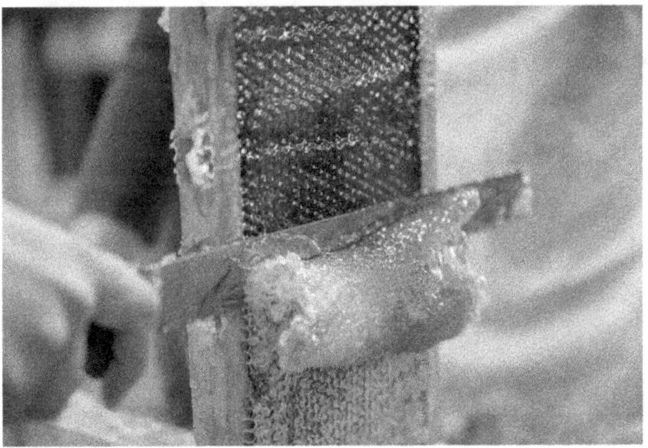

Images showing white comb honey still in the honey frame, and the second showing comb honey being uncapped and ready for extraction.When it comes to pure honey, timing is involved. Therefore it is of great importance for you to understand, or at least have an idea of when honey will be coming in . Most of this information is available on national agriculture or beekeeping websites in your area.

Since it's seasonal, pure honey only comes once,twice or thrice in a year which means you always need to be prepared to stock up on it. You also need a little knowledge on storage(this is not hard since honey can stay well even for 100 years, as long as water or any other substance is not added to it). If it's pure honey that you want, then you need to plan for it. Otherwise, you will be stuck buying honey from convenient stores of which you are not sure of its quality, and where it came from.Working hand in hand with your local beekeeper supplier, means you can pre order, or book to buy a certain amount once its honey flow season. As you wait for the season to approach, you can use the time to save money, so that when the time comes, you have money to buy enough till the next season. In this way you are sure that you always have honey.

Also as long as it's pure and stored well, honey doesn't lose its health properties.

How to Use and Consume honey.

After understanding the type of honey you need and its powerful benefits to your health and wellbeing. Don't just take my word for it. Head out, buy yourself some good natural pure honey, use it regularly (half a jar or 7 spoons a day), take out sugar and gluten. Do this for three months to see how well you improve in health, strength, appearance and even in your relationship with your wife or husband.

After this hit me up and give me a bonus or donate towards my bee projects to help me spread this amazing revelation.

Comb honey

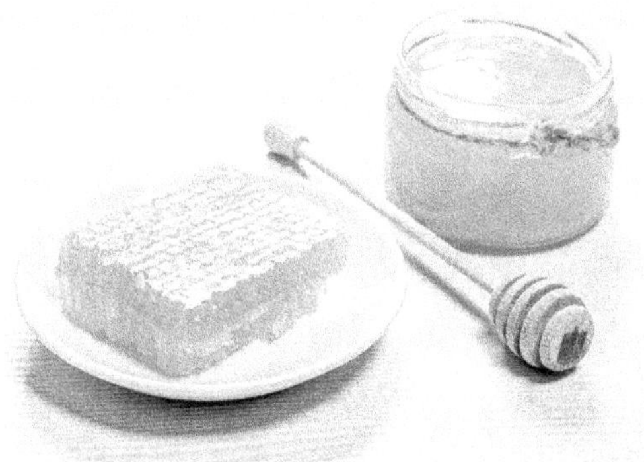

Honey can be eaten directly straight from the hive when still in the combs.

You just bite off a chunk that can fit in your mouth, then simply chew like chewing gum until the sweetness is all gone, then you spit out the empty chewed up comb. Now some honey comb may break withing your mouth as you chew, and you might end up swallowing small bits, but thats ok, it does no harm to your body.

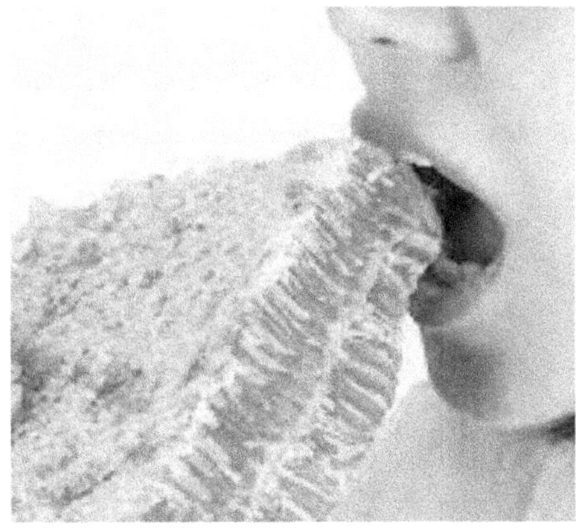

Biting a chunk of comb honey.

LIQUID HONEY IN JARS

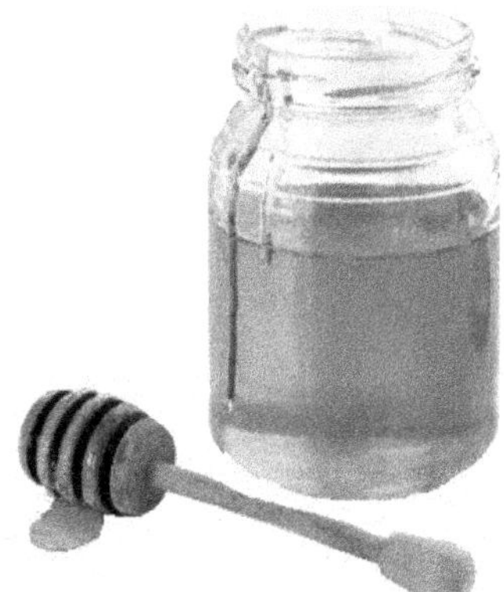

This is perhaps the most common form of which honey is sold and consumed.

Just take up a few spoonfuls for tea instead of sugar. Just remember, to have the tea warm and not hot, so that all the honey properties may remain intact.

Honey can also be used for baking , and cooking however it is good to use it as a topping instead of putting it through heat in the baking process. Heat destroys the natural properties of honey

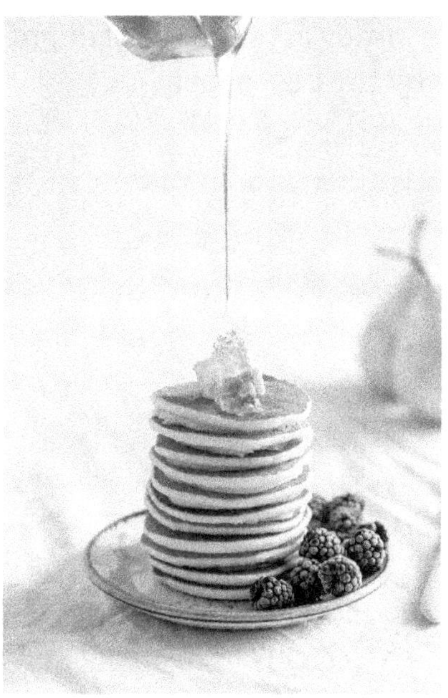

That you can spread over you cake after its baked and cooled or over you salad

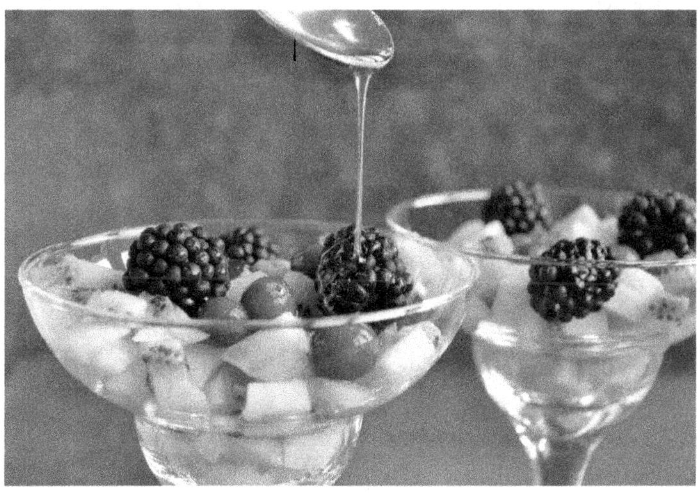

Delicious honey fruit salad.

Crystalized Honey

Crystalized honey in the jar was once liquid.

Depending on the type of nectar, some honey crystallized straight from the hive if not harvested quickly by the beekeeper.

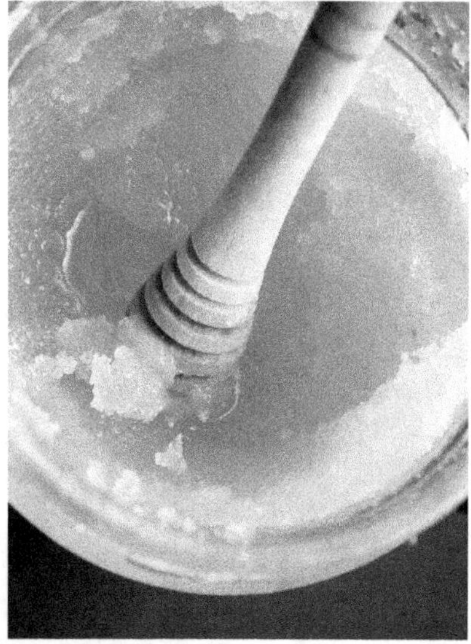

Crystalized honey is easy to scoop up with a spoon and spread over some gluten free bread.

A Simple way is to just take a spoon, and scoop up honey and eat it directly, 7 spoons a day, will keep the doctor away.

Or just do what the cute bear below does, and be happy.

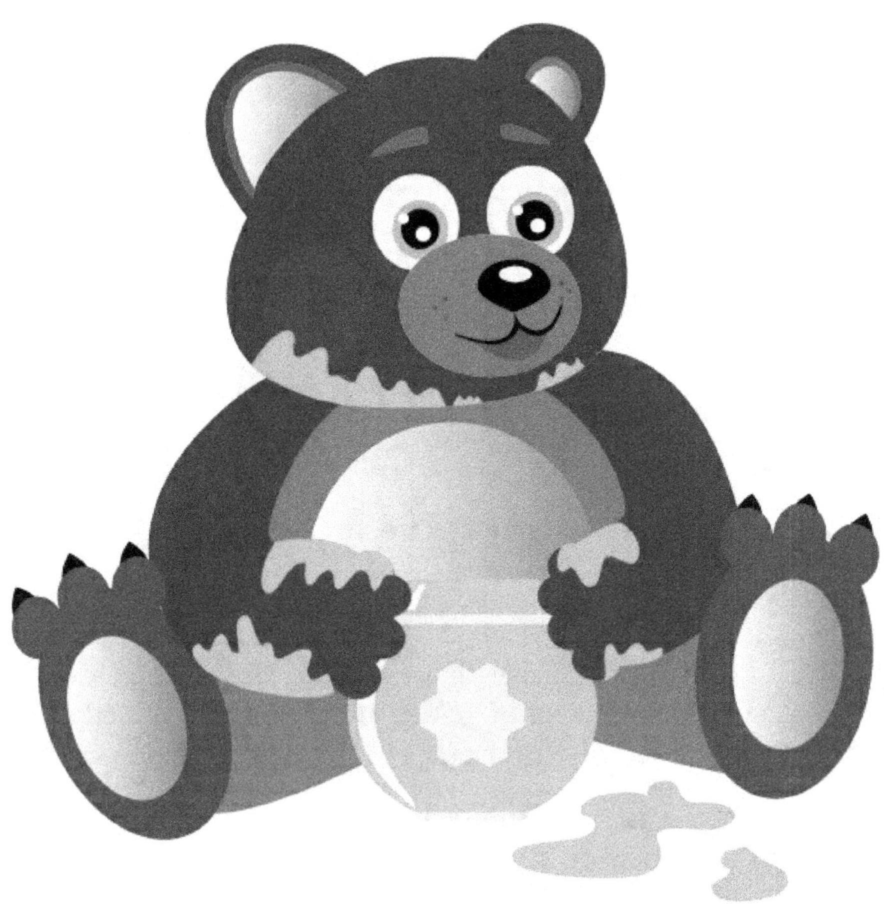

CHAPTER 7: SWEET HARMONY FOR THE BODY AND MIND

Emotional Benefits:

Soothing Sweetness: Honey's Role in Stress Reduction and Quality Sleep

In the midst of life's hustle and bustle, finding moments of tranquility and rest can feel like a distant dream. Yet, nestled within the golden depths of honey lies a natural remedy that offers solace and serenity in the face of stress and sleeplessness.

Honey's ability to calm the mind and promote relaxation is rooted in its rich composition of natural sugars, vitamins, minerals, and amino acids. When consumed, honey triggers the release of serotonin, a neurotransmitter that regulates mood and promotes feelings of well-being. This surge of serotonin not only uplifts the spirits but also helps alleviate stress and anxiety, paving the way for a more peaceful state of mind.

Moreover, honey's unique blend of sugars, including glucose and fructose, serves as a source of sustained energy that helps stabilize blood sugar levels throughout the night. By preventing fluctuations in blood sugar, honey helps maintain a steady flow of energy to the brain during sleep, reducing the likelihood of waking up feeling restless or groggy.

Additionally, honey's natural sweetness stimulates the release of melatonin, the hormone responsible for regulating the sleep-wake cycle. Melatonin levels naturally rise in the evening as darkness falls, signaling to the body that it's time to wind down and prepare for sleep. By consuming honey before bedtime, we can enhance this natural process and promote the onset of restful sleep.

Furthermore, honey's soothing properties extend beyond its nutritional composition to its aromatic profile. The delicate floral notes and warm, comforting aroma of honey evoke feelings of comfort and relaxation, creating a sensory experience that calms the mind and prepares the body for rest.

In essence, honey's calming effect on stress and its role in promoting good sleep offer a natural remedy for the modern afflictions of our fast-paced world. By incorporating honey into our bedtime rituals, whether enjoyed in a warm cup of herbal tea or drizzled over a soothing bowl of oatmeal, we can harness the power of nature to nurture our bodies, calm our minds, and embrace the restorative embrace of sleep.

Holistic Well-Being:

Nurturing the Soul: Honey's Contribution to Emotional and Mental Well-Being

In the whirlwind of modern life, finding moments of peace and contentment can often feel like a distant aspiration. Yet, amidst the chaos, honey emerges as a gentle guardian of emotional and mental well-being, offering solace and nourishment for the soul.

At its core, honey is more than just a sweet indulgence—it's a source of comfort, connection, and joy. The act of savoring honey, whether drizzled over a warm bowl of oatmeal or stirred into a steaming cup of tea, invites us to slow down, savor the moment, and indulge in the simple pleasures of life. In this way, honey becomes a conduit for mindfulness and presence, anchoring us in the here and now and fostering a sense of gratitude and appreciation for life's small delights.

Moreover, honey's natural sweetness has a profound impact on our emotional state, eliciting feelings of warmth, pleasure, and contentment. When consumed, honey triggers the release of serotonin, the "feel-good" neurotransmitter that promotes feelings of happiness and well-being. This surge of serotonin not only uplifts the spirits but also helps alleviate stress and anxiety, creating a sense of inner calm and resilience in the face of life's challenges.

Furthermore, honey's rich aromatic profile and delicate floral notes evoke a sense of comfort and nostalgia, transporting us to simpler times and cherished memories. Whether infused with the scent of wildflowers or the warmth of summer sunshine, honey carries with it the essence of nature's beauty, offering a soothing balm for the soul and a reminder of life's inherent sweetness.

In essence, honey's contribution to overall well-being extends far beyond its nutritional value—it nourishes the heart, uplifts the spirit, and nurtures the soul. By incorporating honey into our daily rituals and savoring its sweetness with intention and mindfulness, we can cultivate a deeper sense of emotional and mental well-being, finding solace and joy in the simple pleasures of life.

CHAPTER 8: THE HEALING SYMPHONY

- **Holistic Healing:**

Holistic Harmony: Honey's Multifaceted Healing Powers

In the realm of natural remedies, few substances rival the multifaceted marvel that is honey. Beyond its delectable sweetness, honey stands as a potent solution of holistic healing, offering a treasure trove of benefits for the body, mind, and spirit.

At the forefront of honey's healing prowess lies its antibacterial and antimicrobial properties, which help combat infections, soothe wounds, and promote tissue regeneration. Whether applied topically to cuts and burns or consumed internally to support immune function, honey serves as a versatile ally in the fight against illness and injury.

Moreover, honey's anti-inflammatory properties work wonders for soothing sore throats, reducing inflammation, and alleviating symptoms of conditions like arthritis and asthma. Its natural antioxidants help neutralize free radicals, protecting cells from oxidative damage and promoting overall health and vitality.

Beyond its physical benefits, honey nurtures emotional well-being, offering comfort and solace in times of stress and anxiety. Its natural sweetness triggers the release of serotonin, promoting feelings of happiness and relaxation. The act of savoring honey becomes a ritual of self-care, grounding us in the present moment and fostering a sense of calm and contentment.

Furthermore, honey's rich aromatic profile and delicate floral notes stimulate the senses, evoking memories, and emotions that uplift the spirit and nourish the soul. Its warm, comforting embrace serves as a reminder of nature's abundance and the interconnectedness of all living things.

In essence, honey's holistic healing properties transcend the boundaries of conventional medicine, offering a holistic approach to health and well-being that encompasses the body, mind, and spirit. By embracing honey as a natural remedy and incorporating it into our daily lives, we can tap into its transformative power and cultivate a harmonious balance of health and vitality.

Chapter 9: The Rising Demand for Honey

- **Market Challenges:**

Navigating the Sweet Dilemma: Challenges in Preserving Honey Purity Amidst Rising Demand

As the allure of honey continues to captivate palates worldwide, a bittersweet dilemma emerges: the challenge of maintaining purity in the face of soaring demand. While honey's popularity is a testament to its timeless appeal and myriad benefits, the rising demand presents a host of challenges for beekeepers, producers, and consumers alike.

One of the primary challenges in preserving honey purity stems from the pressure to meet growing market demand while maintaining ethical and sustainable beekeeping practices. With increased demand comes the temptation to cut corners, leading to practices such as feeding bees sugar syrup or diluting honey with cheaper additives. These shortcuts not only compromise the quality and authenticity of the honey but also undermine the integrity of the entire industry.

Furthermore, the global nature of the honey market complicates efforts to ensure purity and traceability. With honey sourced from diverse regions around the world, it becomes increasingly difficult to verify the origin and quality of each batch. This lack of transparency opens the door to adulteration and fraud, as unscrupulous producers seek to capitalize on the high demand for honey by passing off inferior products as genuine.

Moreover, environmental factors such as climate change and habitat loss pose additional challenges to honey purity. As bee populations decline and floral resources dwindle, bees are forced to forage over greater distances, increasing the risk of contamination from pesticides, pollutants, and other environmental stressors. These external pressures not only threaten the health and well-being of bees but also compromise the purity and safety of the honey they produce.

In the face of these challenges, preserving honey purity requires a concerted effort from all stakeholders in the honey industry. Beekeepers must uphold strict standards of ethical beekeeping and sustainable practices, ensuring the health and welfare of their bee colonies. Producers and regulators must implement rigorous testing and certification protocols to verify the authenticity and quality of honey products. And consumers must remain vigilant and discerning, choosing reputable sources and demanding transparency in labeling and sourcing.

In essence, maintaining honey purity amidst rising demand is a complex and multifaceted endeavor that requires collaboration, innovation, and unwavering commitment to the principles of integrity and sustainability. By working together to overcome these challenges, we can ensure that honey continues to be cherished as nature's golden gift—a pure and precious treasure to be savored and enjoyed for generations to come.

- **Consumer Vigilance:**

The Golden Standard: Why Consumer Vigilance is Key in Ensuring Honey Quality

In a marketplace brimming with options, the quest for quality has never been more vital, especially when it comes to honey—the golden elixir of nature. As consumers, our vigilance plays a crucial role in upholding the integrity and purity of this beloved commodity.

At the heart of the matter lies the need to distinguish between genuine, high-quality honey and its lesser counterparts. Genuine honey, sourced from ethical beekeepers and produced through sustainable practices, offers a wealth of health benefits and sensory delights. Conversely, adulterated or low-quality honey, tainted by additives or inferior ingredients, not only fails to deliver on its promises but also undermines consumer trust and compromises health and well-being.

Consumer vigilance is essential in safeguarding against the myriad forms of honey adulteration and fraud that pervade the market. From dilution with sugar syrups to the addition of artificial flavorings and preservatives, the methods employed by unscrupulous producers are as diverse as they are deceptive. By scrutinizing labels, verifying certifications, and patronizing reputable producers, consumers can empower themselves to make informed choices and protect themselves against deception and disappointment.

Moreover, consumer vigilance serves as a powerful force for change within the honey industry, driving demand for transparency, accountability, and ethical practices. By demanding honesty and integrity from producers and regulators alike, consumers can help elevate standards of quality and ensure that genuine, high-quality honey remains the gold standard in the marketplace.

In essence, the importance of consumer vigilance in safeguarding honey quality cannot be overstated. By remaining vigilant, informed, and discerning, consumers can champion the purity and integrity of honey, ensuring that each spoonful is a true taste of nature's bounty—a sweet symphony of health, pleasure, and authenticity.

Conclusion: A Life Sweetened

- **Reflecting on Transformation:**

Reflecting on the transformative power of honey in my life, I am in awe of the profound impact this humble natural remedy has had on my well-being. Despite the challenges posed by dietary sensitivities and health issues like acne Keloidalis nuchae and asthma, honey emerged as a steadfast ally, shielding me from harm and guiding me toward a path of healing and vitality.

In the face of gluten-induced distress and the threat of chronic diseases, honey stood as a beacon of hope, offering relief and protection where conventional remedies fell short. Its antibacterial, anti-inflammatory, and immune-boosting properties became my lifeline, fortifying my body and spirit against the onslaught of illness and discomfort.

Through the simple act of incorporating honey into my daily routine, I witnessed a profound transformation take place—a transformation marked by newfound strength, resilience, and inner peace. With each spoonful of honey, I felt the healing embrace of nature's bounty, soothing my ailments and restoring balance to my body and soul.

In the journey of life, honey has been more than just a sweet indulgence—it has been a source of nourishment, empowerment, and inspiration. Its transformative power knows no bounds, transcending the limitations of science and medicine to touch every aspect of my being with its golden touch.

As I look back on my journey with honey, I am filled with gratitude for the profound impact it has had on my life. Through its gentle yet potent Power, honey has not only healed my body but also awakened within me a deeper appreciation for the wonders of nature and the infinite possibilities that lie within each drop of this precious solution. Truly, the transformative power of honey is a testament to the enduring beauty and wisdom of the natural world—a gift that I will forever cherish and hold dear.

- **Enduring Value:**

In a world filled with processed foods and artificial additives, the enduring value of embracing pure, raw honey as a daily ally shines brightly like a beacon of authenticity and wholesomeness. Beyond its exquisite taste and golden hue, pure honey offers a myriad of health benefits, nourishing the body, mind, and soul with its rich array of nutrients and healing properties.

As we navigate the complexities of modern living, pure, raw honey stands as a steadfast companion, offering comfort, sustenance, and vitality in equal measure. From its antibacterial and antioxidant properties to its ability to soothe stress and promote restful sleep, honey is a natural remedy that transcends time and tradition—a testament to the enduring wisdom of nature's bounty.

In embracing pure, raw honey as a daily ally, we honor the legacy of generations past who revered this precious solution for its healing powers and cherished it as a symbol of abundance and resilience. With each spoonful, we connect with the rhythms of the natural world, savoring the sweetness of life and celebrating the timeless wisdom of the honeybee.

So let us raise our jars to the humble honeybee and the golden treasure it bestows upon us. Let us savor each drop of pure, raw honey as a reminder of our connection to the earth and to each other. And let us embrace the enduring value of this sweet ally, knowing that in its purity lies the promise of health, happiness, and harmony for generations to come.

Thank you for the time you have taken to both purchase and read this book.
My only joy is to hear that the information you have received from this has done great in your life and led you to great health.

This topic about honey is huge. I encourage you to also do more research while being skeptical. Also feel free to reach out to me through the social media links below for more guidance .
Be blessed.

You can reach out to me for other great health books, comments, concerns, appreciation messages or simply to donate and support my work through the links below.

Links and Social media
https://www.remedyscout.com/

https://www.facebook.com/remedyscout

https://www.youtube.com/channel/
UC5v2LxY2TJQRluJejf_jOHQ

https://remedyscout.gumroad.com/l/icehgh?

EMMANUEL LUBANGAKENE

fbclid=IwAR3IvmQ7WPXkZWiIauNkQy8zS6I4aG_r-
xUbTOJdZGjlgXgovWYKB6ZPzBA

emmkene@gmail.com